The Little Book
of Health for

Men

Boosting life's potential

Sharon Platt-McDonald
MSc RHV RM RGN

First published 2010

© 2010 The Stanborough Press Ltd

British Library Cataloguing in Publication Data.
A catalogue record for this book is available from the
British Library.

ISBN 1-904685-87-0

Published by The Stanborough Press Ltd,
Grantham, Lincolnshire.

Designed by Abigail Murphy

Printed in Thailand.

Take responsibility for your health

In this volume men's health issues are put under the microscope. As you read, you will hopefully find something that connects with your health needs or particular area of interest. If you are already on a well-established path to health, it is my hope that this encourages you to keep going, as it will pay dividends for the future. If health has been an area of challenge, may you be inspired to rediscover the steps to good health and place wellbeing on your daily agenda.

Professor Alan White, chairman of the Men's Health Forum, states that although it is important for men to take responsibility for their own health, an area to be addressed is the availability and access to health services. It is these aspects that sometimes preclude men from seeking the necessary help in a timely manner. Christine Hancock, director of the Oxford Health Alliance, adds, 'If you think that nearly 14 million men work full-time and of those 28% are working over 45 hours, then getting to the services is actually very problematic.'

Workplaces seeking to address this issue are now providing health screening for their employees. In addition, however, it is recognised that more information specific to men's health should be readily available in a variety of formats to engage their interest.

This book is packed with health nuggets, tips and tools to advise you how to preserve your health and wellbeing, and gives insights into knowing when to seek help. As you embrace the information, enjoy the journey to enhanced health and wellbeing.
You are worth it!

Sharon

'Life is about more than just maintaining oneself, it is about extending oneself. Otherwise living is only not dying.'
Simone de Beauvoir

Physical wellbeing

Physical activity

Research demonstrates that exercise or lack of it is more a determinant of health than people give credit for. In fact, exercise can lengthen life. Studies show that regular exercise (most days of the week) can enhance overall wellbeing and reduce the risk of certain cancers.

Several studies have pointed to the positive impact of exercise on the body's cardiovascular system. One large study over a 15-year period found a correlation between men who exercised and the healthier levels of blood pressure and lower stroke risk compared with those who did not exercise. The research revealed that the physically active men were 57% less likely to develop high blood pressure. Another study demonstrated that physically active people had 68% fewer strokes than those who were inactive.

Breaking the sedentary habit

Here are a few tips to help increase your level of activity even when doing domestic and work activities.

At home:

- Walk around while talking on the phone.

- If you have an exercise bike, pedal while watching television or phoning.

- While reading or in a seated position make circular movements with your toes.

- Stand up for 10 minutes in every hour if watching TV for a lengthy period.

- Turn the channels manually rather than using the remote.

- Increase the pace while doing chores. You can turn gardening into a mini fitness routine by raking leaves vigorously, turning over the soil and so on.

At work:

• Take the stairs instead of the lift as it burns more calories by increasing your metabolism.

• Utilise break times to take short walks.

• Don't eat lunch at your desk. Lunch at least five minutes away from your place of work so you can take a brisk walk.

Out and about:

• Park a good distance away from
your destination in order to
increase your steps per day.

• When travelling on public transport, stand
on the bus or train. This burns an extra
70 calories for every hour of travelling.

• Use stairs rather than lifts or escalators.
If using escalators, walk up them.

Exercise update

While outdoor exercise has its advantages,
pollution could be a deterrent for joggers. A
recent study by the University of Edinburgh
found that exposure to diesel fumes could
cause blood clots which in turn puts pressure
on the heart, making heart attack or stroke
more likely. Scientists are now advising us to
exercise away from traffic jams to avoid
pollution. Parkland areas are less polluted
and have softer surfaces, causing
less stress on the bones.

Plan effective physical activity

The most effective exercises for men are those which combine the elements of building strength, endurance and flexibility. From these three key aspects, physical activity is divided into three main groups of exercises. They should incorporate the following: aerobics for cardiovascular workouts, weights for building strength, stretching to increase flexibility and supple limbs.

Physical activity tips

The following **age-related fitness
programme** is a suggested exercise
plan relative to your age.

• Work out at least three times a week with a
rest day between each workout.

• Other physical activities (like walking) can still
be undertaken in between workouts to achieve
the recommended level of physical activity on
between 5 and 6 days a week.

Twenties

Focus: Concentrate on resilience through aggressive play, for example basketball.

Strength training: 30 minutes three times a week doing three sets from each exercise group.

Aerobic training: 15-20 minutes three times a week – 80-85% maximum heart rate.

Stretching: 5 minutes during each workout.

Advice/caution: Protect shoulders and knees.

Thirties

Focus: Take more time on aerobic activities (like swimming) for overall body workout and cardiovascular health.

Strength training: 20 minutes three times a week doing two sets from each exercise group.

Aerobic training: 30 minutes three times a week – 70% maximum heart rate.

Stretching: 5-10 minutes during each workout.

Advice/caution: Commence slowly until limits are defined.

Forties

Focus: Undertake moderate strength training.

Strength training: 20 minutes twice a week with two sets from each exercise group. Use lighter weights on the third day for 45 minutes. Include circuit training.

Aerobic training: 25 minutes twice a week – 60-70% maximum heart rate. 30 minutes light activity two more days a week.

Stretching: 5-10 minutes during each workout.

Advice/caution: Increase abdominal exercises to tackle any bulging midriff.

Fifties plus

Focus: Concentrate on weight-bearing exercises like brisk walking to keep bones strong and healthy.

Strength training: 20 minutes twice a week. 45 minutes circuit training once a week.

Aerobic training: 20 minutes twice a week – 60-70% maximum heart rate. Brisk walking two other days a week.

Stretching: 5-10 minutes during each workout.

Advice/caution: Reduce pressure or stress on joints and back.

(Adapted from *Healthy Living Guide* – Exercise and Health)

Physique

If you observe an unwanted bulge around your middle and would like to tame the spreading girth, then read on.

Four 'must dos' for a flatter stomach:

• Cut down on fats in your diet. This means grilling, steaming, baking and poaching instead of frying. Switch to a low-fat diet with a higher volume of fresh fruits and vegetables and whole grains. Your carbohydrates should include whole wheat, oats, rye, millet and so on instead of white flour.

• Commence abdominal exercises – stomach crunches, press-ups, squats, leg and knee raises and so on. If you are looking for washboard abs then a regular intense total abdominal workout programme is best – via good men's health magazines or joining a gym.

• Try fat-burning aerobic exercises like jogging, badminton, squash, tennis, swimming or rowing.

• Be conscious of posture. Stand up straight and regularly pull in your stomach muscles. This will eventually become a subconscious action. Toned abdominal muscles enhance posture, and vice versa.

Why weight matters

The health risk of being overweight has been well documented over the years. The more overweight, the greater the risk. Reports indicate that if you are more than 20% above your optimal weight, or have a BMI (Body Mass Index) of above 30, you are considered obese and at high risk of serious health problems. However, girth measurements are now used more accurately to assess body weight and health implications.

Here are some of the dangers you might face if you are overweight:

- Twice the risk of high blood pressure. This increases to nearly six times the risk if you are over 45.

- Increased risk of developing adult onset diabetes.

- Risk of high cholesterol leading to blocked arteries.

- Increased risk of heart disease and heart attack.

- Higher risk of stroke.

- Increased risk of cancers of the colon and prostate.

- More likely to experience sleep apnoea.

- Higher incidence of osteoarthritis, gall bladder disease and sexual problems.

- Shorter life span.

Overweight?

Don't worry. Just increasing your level of activity and adjusting eating habits will produce positive changes in your weight.

However, if you suffer from an endocrine disorder which slows your metabolism, your GP or health practitioner may be able to advise you on important steps to take in order to manage your weight.

In order to lose weight you need to burn more calories than you're consuming. That means you need to increase output in terms of activity and decrease input in terms of food portions and calories. The recommended suggestions for men are to undertake the following:

• Always eat breakfast. Skipping breakfast increases weight gain, because the body requires nourishment after a night without food and when it does not get it the metabolic system slows down as it tries to hold on to nutrients.

• Reduce daily calorie intake by about 500 calories.

• Increase fibre in the diet which gives a feeling of fullness and prevents snacking. Try sweet potatoes which are higher in fibre than regular potatoes.

• Eat complex carbohydrates. These are whole-grain starchy foods made from whole wheat, rolled oats, barley, rye, millet and found in whole-wheat pasta, brown rice, whole-wheat bread. These foods are nourishing and have a low glycaemic index. Simple carbohydrates like white flour and processed sugary foods have a high glycaemic index which causes a surge in blood sugar levels, resulting in high output of insulin to cope with raised blood sugars.

• Avoid processed food which is generally less nourishing.

• Have less sugar, fat and salt.

• If you need to snack, then choose fruit rather than biscuits, crisps, chocolates or sweets.

• Avoid alcohol.

• Exercise for at least 30 minutes a minimum of five days a week. Choose activities that assist all-over muscle toning and cardiovascular support such as brisk walking, running, swimming, cycling or rowing. If you are very overweight then a specific exercise programme may be needed to ensure you build up slowly without putting your body under excess strain.

A realistic goal is to aim to lose 1-2lbs each week.

You can do it!

Recent research has indicated one area where men beat women in health matters – flab fighting! Men can control their food cravings better than women, thus increasing their chances of winning the battle with the bulge. Brain scans reveal that men have far less activity in the part of the brain that controls desire for food, which may be the reason why men may find it easier to lose weight by simply 'turning off' their thoughts of food and so are more disciplined in handling food choices.

Good night

The *New Scientist* published a study on the impact of sleep deficit. It was found that men who have disturbed sleep suffer more health deficits than women. Also men suffer from significantly disturbed sleep when they share a bed. Getting a good night's sleep is essential.

Stress level and mental capacity were tested. Although women also had disturbed sleep when sharing a bed, they slept more deeply and their stress levels and mental scores did not reveal the deficits indicated in the results for males.

It was found, however, that natural remedies produced more enhanced sleep and encouraged couples to sleep better in the same bed.

The following natural remedies were found to be beneficial:

• Valerian. Various studies have shown this herbal supplement can help ease insomnia.

• Chamomile tea. Sipping this drink before bedtime can aid relaxation and, therefore, induce sleep.

• Lavender. A few drops of essential oil of lavender on your pillow creates not only a pleasant aroma but is also reported to aid relaxation.

Cardiovascular health

Blood pressure

A study of men with normal blood pressure levels found variation in the readings according to the level of activity that the men engaged in. The physically active men were 57% less likely to develop high blood pressure during the 15-years follow-up study compared to men who were sedentary. Another study demonstrated that physically active men had 68% fewer strokes.

Anger and disease

Researchers have looked at the impact of anger on the heart. Controlling anger has a beneficial health impact. Men who regularly exhibit angry behaviours are nearly 20% more likely to develop heart disease than men who have a less aggressive approach. Men who already have heart disease and give way to angry outbursts are 24% more likely to have a heart attack or stroke than men who are able to use other forms of expression like meditation and exercise as an outlet for stress.

Health aware

More than 100,000 men in the UK die prematurely each year because they neglect their health! Men are more reluctant to lead healthy lifestyles than women and also, crucially, they are much less likely to visit their GP, so early symptoms of disease are less likely to be picked up. One way of keeping your health in check is by attending your GP's surgery on an annual basis for health checks.

Key health checks

Prostate-specific antigen (PSA) test. This test, key to detecting prostate cancer, measures the amount of PSA in the blood. If the PSA level is high, it may indicate the presence of cancer cells.

Digital rectal examination. The doctor inserts a gloved finger into the rectum and feels the prostate through the wall of the rectum. Any hard or lumpy areas are suspicious and may be a sign of cancer. In the UK and US, prostate cancer is the most common cancer in men over age 65.

Sigmoidoscopy. The doctor uses a thin, flexible tube with a light at the end to look inside the lower part of the colon and rectum for growths or abnormal areas. Studies show that a sigmoidoscopy once every five years has saved lives.

Colonoscopy. This is similar to a sigmoidoscopy, but this test looks at the whole colon. Some doctors now recommend a colonoscopy every ten years, as the incidence of colorectal cancer appears to be increasing.

Cancer

Cancer facts for men

Cancer Research UK lists the following as the most common cancers in men:

• Prostate cancer is the most common cancer in men in the UK. More than 35,000 men per annum in the UK are diagnosed with prostate cancer.

• Prostate cancer is the second most common cause of cancer death in UK men. Each year around 10,200 men in the UK die from prostate cancer.

• Lung cancer is the second most common cancer in men, with more than 22,300 new cases diagnosed in the UK each year.

• Around 20,400 men are diagnosed with bowel cancer in the UK each year, making it the third most common cancer in men.

• Around 2,100 men are diagnosed with testicular cancer every year in the UK, and rates appear to be rising.

• Testicular cancer represents only 1% of all cancers in men, but it is the single biggest cause of cancer-related deaths in men aged 15 to 35 years in the UK.

A BBC report (quoting data from Cancer Research UK) found that men are 16% more likely to develop cancer and 40% more likely to die from cancer than women. The BBC stated, 'There is no known biological reason for this but it may be because women take better care of themselves.' The report suggested that men are more reluctant to lead healthy lifestyles than women.

Cancer risk

Did you know?

• About 75% of adults in England are not
eating the recommended five portions of fruit
and vegetables each day which research
demonstrates as beneficial in
lowering cancer risk.

• A high intake of red and processed meat will
increase your chances of developing bowel
cancer, whereas a diet rich in fibre
will reduce your risk.

• Obesity and being overweight is linked to at
least 10% of colon cancers in the UK.

• Exercise reduces cancer risks. Cancer Research UK found that 30 minutes of moderate activity a day, five days a week, can have a positive effect on your health.

• Research demonstrates that an inactive lifestyle increases risk of bowel cancer.

• Research has shown that people drinking more than 30g a day of alcohol (around 4 units) have an increased risk of bowel cancer.

Prostate cancer

- It is the most common cancer in men in the UK and is on the increase.

- One man dies of prostate cancer every hour in the UK.

- Most cases of prostate cancer occur in men over 50, and more than 70% of cases are in men over 65.

- Having one or more close relatives with prostate cancer also increases a man's risk of developing it.

- West Africans and Caribbeans are significantly more likely than white men to develop prostate cancer and are more likely to die from it.

- Men born in Asia have a lower risk of prostate cancer than men born in the UK.

If detected early, prostate cancer can be treated. It can usually be detected in its early stages by a blood test called prostate-specific antigen (PSA) and a digital rectal examination.

Risk of prostate cancer increases with age, so it is rare to find this cancer in men under 50. Cancer Research UK estimates that by the age of 80, more than half of men have cancerous changes in their prostate. Due to the slow growth of prostate cancer, many are unaware that they have the disease and may die of unrelated causes.

Signs and symptoms

Since an enlarged prostate can cause the same symptoms as prostate cancer, it is best to seek medical advice promptly. This is because both benign and malignant tumours in this region cause significant pressure, press on the urethra and block the flow of urine.

Subsequently the following
symptoms can be experienced:

• Difficulty in passing urine

• Sudden urge to urinate and having
to rush to the toilet to pass urine

• Passing urine more often than
usual, especially at night

• Pain on passing urine (less common)

• Blood in the urine or semen (less common)

Other symptoms of prostate cancer

Usually cancer of the prostate gland grows slowly, especially in older men. This generally produces mild symptoms which occur over many years. As the symptom may appear mild to the sufferer he may not seek medical help promptly. As a result, unfortunately sometimes the first symptoms of prostate are from prostate cancer cells which have spread to the bones.

This may cause pain in the
bones in the following areas:

- Back

- Hips

- Pelvis

- Other bony areas

Preventive factors

• It has been found that men who have a high consumption of tomatoes reduce their risk of prostate cancer by 40%. Lycopene in tomatoes is an important nutrient and powerful antioxidant with the ability to quench or neutralise free radicals which are organic molecules responsible for ageing, tissue damage and diseases.

• Several studies have also demonstrated that the herbal supplement saw palmetto can improve prostate health.

• There is a link between diet and prostate cancer. A low-fat diet of only 12% of the daily calories coming from fat (as opposed to our usual 35-40%) could cut the rate of prostate cancer.

• The Prostate Cancer Charity recommends increasing the intake of cruciferous vegetables such as broccoli, snacking on a handful of Brazil nuts daily and including omega-3-rich foods in the diet.

• A study published in the *British Journal of Urology International* found that men in their 50s who had sexual intercourse more than 10 times a month gained some protection. The research concluded that hormones or toxins that may lead to cancerous changes may be released from the male during lovemaking, thus reducing the risk of prostate cancer.

• A report presented to the American Urological Association identified that men previously treated for prostate cancer were significantly less likely to develop more cancerous growth by drinking pomegranate juice.

Testicular cancer

- Currently, about 1,500 men a year (around 1 in 400) develop the disease in the UK.

- The number of UK cases has trebled in the past 25 years and is still rising.

- Testicular cancer is most common in men aged 15 to 45.

Although testicular cancer is rare, it is not at all uncommon to find a lump in your testicles. There are many conditions that can be easily confused with testicular cancer, but it is best to get checked, just to be sure.

Cancer Research UK advises regular monthly testicular self-examination.

The following signs should be checked for:

- a lump detected in one testicle

- pain and tenderness in either testicle

- an increase in size of a testicle (one is normally larger than the other but the size and shape should remain more or less the same)

- a build-up of fluid inside the scrotum

- a dull ache in the abdomen or groin

- a heavy or dragging feeling in the groin or scrotum

- discharge or pus from the penis

- blood in the sperm at ejaculation

If you perform a self-examination and find a lump, you are advised to go to your doctor.

Risk factors

The cause of testicular cancer is yet to be fully established. Studies on how to prevent it are ongoing. There are certain risk factors that can increase your chance of getting testicular cancer. These are:

• Age: Diagnosis of testicular cancer is made more frequently in the young and middle-aged than in elderly men.

• Un-descended testes at birth: This condition may increase the risk of testicular cancer by as much as five to ten times.

• Inherited genetic factors may play a role in up to 20% of testicular cancers.

• Family history: The risk of developing this cancer is increased if you have a father, brother or son who has had testicular cancer.

• Previous testicular cancer: A previous diagnosis of testicular cancer increases the risk of developing cancer in the other testicle.

• Race and ethnicity: Testicular cancer is most common in Caucasian (white) men. It is rare in non-Caucasian populations with the exception of New Zealand Maori.

Regular self-examination will help you become more aware of the normal feel and size of your testicles so that you can spot any abnormalities early.

Prostatism/Benign prostatic hypertrophy (BPH)

This condition occurs when the prostate gland begins to enlarge. The prostate gland is situated at the base of the bladder around the urethra (tube that urine passes through). This organ is about the size of a walnut and makes the liquid (semen) that carries sperm on ejaculation. Protastism (enlarged prostate) is considered a non-cancerous condition and is in fact termed as benign prostatic hyperplasia or hypertrophy (BPH).

Incidence

The condition usually occurs once men reach their 40s and their prostate gland starts to enlarge. It is estimated that one in four men in their 50s and one in two men over 60 will experience to some degree the discomforts of an enlarged prostate.

This does not cause a problem for some men. Others experience significant discomfort and great inconvenience.

Common symptoms

- having to get up throughout the night to pass water

- urgency of urine – having to find a toilet urgently when out and sometimes not making it in time

- difficulty passing urine

- a weak, irregular stream

- dribbling after passing urine

- incomplete emptying of the bladder and feeling the bladder isn't empty

- continually needing to go to the toilet

Some or all of these symptoms may be
experienced due to an enlarged prostate.
Additionally, the annoyance of disturbed sleep
patterns for the sufferer and his spouse
can bring its own health hazards
of sleep deprivation.

Men should not hesitate to see their doctor
who will be able to offer the most
appropriate intervention.

Treatment options

• For minor symptoms it is usual to employ only lifestyle changes. This entails encouraging foods like red tomatoes and soya and cutting down on foods high in fat, caffeine and alcohol which have been found to impact the prostate negatively.

• For more moderate symptoms, your doctor may prescribe medication specifically to shrink the size of the prostate in order to relieve the symptoms.

• For more persistent and painful symptoms which do not respond to dietary changes and prescription medicine an operation is advised.

• Saw palmetto. This natural remedy has become the first over-the-counter prostate treatment to win a UK herbal medicine licence. Trials have found that taking saw palmetto following diagnosis could help delay enlargement of the prostate and prevent surgery. It's worth speaking with your GP about herbal remedies, especially this one.

Sexual health

Impotence

Impotence is now more commonly known as erectile dysfunction (ED). This condition occurs when men find they are unable to achieve or sustain an erection adequate for sexual intercourse.

ED facts

• Erectile dysfunction is a problem for at least one in every ten men in the UK.

• Half of all men aged over 40 have trouble getting an erection at least once.

• A significant proportion of men experience some degree of impotence at some point.

• Some men experience guilt, anger or depression as a result. Others lose interest in sex and relationships may become strained.

- It is advised that if erectile problems persist for several weeks, medical advice should be sought, as the cause could be an underlying health condition.

- Lifestyle changes, such as losing weight and exercise, can correct the problem.

- Some men may need medication such as sildenafil (known as Viagra).

General causes and risk factors

• Around 70% of erectile dysfunction has physical causes and 30% psychological causes. However, some men experience both physical and psychological reasons for the condition.

• Most men experience occasions at some time in their lives when they cannot achieve or sustain an erection, as a result of fatigue, stress or excessive alcohol consumption.

• The most common physiological cause is atherosclerosis – caused by fatty deposits which damage or clog the small blood vessels which control blood supply to the penis.

• Psychological problems may also impact ED. These may include stress, anxiety, depression, relationship problems or other serious ongoing challenges.

Age-related causes

• In younger men, ED is often caused by anxiety. This mostly relates to nervousness about having sex, pleasing their partner or causing an unplanned pregnancy.

• In middle age, stress, overwork and tiredness are often factors.

• Among older men, physical causes become more common. These include diseases such as diabetes and heart disease, thyroid or kidney problems, high blood pressure, damage to nerves or blood vessels, pelvic surgery or trauma, heavy smoking and medication side-effects.

Interventions

Treatment commences with taking the first step to talk to someone qualified to deal with health and sexual problems. This could be your GP or a specialist in this area. An assessment will then be undertaken which includes a check to look for physical causes, advice on possible treatments and referral to a suitable therapist if appropriate.

Communication with a patient and sensitive spouse will help in the recovery process but sometimes sexual counselling may be necessary.

Medication

There has been a radical change in the treatment of ED in the past decade. Relatively new oral medicines have emerged which assist men in achieving an erection. Generally these drugs have worked for the majority of men, whether the cause was physiological or psychological. However some of the popular medications do not suit everyone and can cause significant side effects. Other treatment options are mechanical aids such as vacuum pumps or penile implants, intra-urethral pellet therapy and injections into the penis.

Lifestyle changes

To reduce risk of ED:

• Avoid smoking and alcohol.

• Eat healthily – reduce fats, salt, sugar and processed foods and opt for natural products and fresh foods.

• Take regular exercise.

• Relax more and enjoy social events.

- Get plenty of rest.

- Manage stress effectively.

- Have a good work-life balance.

Advice and support – Sexual Dysfunction
Association Helpline: 0870 774 3571
Email: *info@sda.uk.net*
Website: *www.sda.uk.net*

Natural remedies

Men who are worried about the side effects of conventional medication like Viagra are turning to other forms of intervention with some success. Trials have been carried out on various herbal remedies. The University of Milan published a report which revealed that the Chinese herb called horny goat weed has an active ingredient which produces similar results to Viagra. The scientists modified a compound in the plant called *icariin* and found that its efficacy was similar to Viagra.

A study by Dr Steven Lamm found that horny goat weed had testosterone-like effects which included increased blood flow to the penile region, increased sperm production, stimulated sensory nerves and increased sexual desire, activity and stamina.

All natural remedies can have side effects. If you have health conditions, discuss any alternative medicines or therapies with your health practitioner first.

Anyone experiencing sexual problems such as erectile dysfunction should consult his GP as this can sometimes be a symptom of other conditions such as heart disease or diabetes.

Emotional wellbeing

Be happy

Laughter is medicine. Scientists have found
that adults laugh on average 15 times a day,
while children laugh around 400 times daily.
When we indulge in play and laughter, the
laughter releases chemicals in the brain called
endorphins (also called happy hormones)
which relax muscles and relieve pain.
They also help as stress busters.

Stress impact

Studies show equal numbers of men and women complaining of stress. However, they are stressed by different things and react in different ways.

Stressors for men

Peter Baker, editor of *malehealth.co.uk*, states, 'Stress is not just about having a hyperactive lifestyle. Having no role and being hard up is very stressful too.'

Unemployment – loss of self-esteem, financial difficulties.

Work changes – outsourcing, longer hours, temporary contracts.

Changing roles – not main breadwinner.

Modern man – Society now expects men to devote more time to home and family as well as work. Subsequently after working long hours men feel pressured to be domesticated, entertain the children and be ideal partners.

How men cope

Men are less likely than women to talk about how they feel and seek help from a doctor or anyone else. Most men wait until medical symptoms of stress emerge, such as chest pains, headaches and stomach problems, before visiting their GP. They tend to choose escape routes like exercise, drinking, smoking or driving aggressively.

Mind reports three-quarters of suicides in the UK are by men. Men suffer equally from depression as women, but are less likely to be diagnosed by a doctor.

Reports indicate that men and women benefit equally from effective stress management. As effective are good time management and better work-life balance. Other therapeutic interventions like exercise, prayerful reflection, deep breathing, massage, listening to relaxing music, have also been found to be beneficial.

Anxiety linked to dementia in men

A recent UK study highlighted the link between current emotional wellbeing and a predictor of mental wellbeing in later life. The study was undertaken with a cohort of 1,481 men aged 48 to 67 years at baseline anxiety assessment level and measured cognition 17 years later. The researchers found that those with high anxiety levels at baseline were significantly more likely to develop dementia. This report does not establish a causal link but strongly suggests that managing stress and anxiety positively may influence quality of life in the later years.

Depression in men

Depression is a loaded word. People tend, wrongly, to associate it with weakness and excessive emotion. This is especially true with men. Depressed men are less likely than women to acknowledge feelings of self-loathing and hopelessness. Instead, they tend to complain about fatigue, irritability, sleep problems and loss of interest in work and hobbies. Symptoms of depression in men include anger, aggression, violence, reckless behaviour and substance abuse. Even though depression rates for women are twice as high as those in men, men are a higher suicide risk, especially older men.

Common signs and symptoms of depression

• Loss of interest in life activities. Decreased interest in daily activities, no interest in or ability to enjoy social activities, hobbies or sexual intimacy.

• Poor concentration. Difficulty focusing, making decisions or remembering things (typically short-term memory).

• Feelings of helplessness and hopelessness. A mindset that sees only challenges. Having a bleak outlook which expresses the view that things will not get better and an inability to impact or improve the situation.

• Altered sleep patterns. Insomnia – difficulty getting to sleep or waking in the early hours. Oversleeping (hypersomnia) may be another indicator.

• Appetite or weight changes. Increased or decreased appetite. Significant weight loss or weight gain – for example a change of more than 5% of body weight in a month.

• Loss of energy. Constantly feeling fatigued and drained, no matter how much rest one gets.

• Neurological and physical changes. Nervousness, anxiety, irritability, worry and/or physical symptoms such as sluggishness, palpitations, headaches, cramps or aches and pains that do not ease with treatment.

• Self-loathing. This includes negative self-talk and highlights perceived faults and mistakes as major character flaws. Experiences strong feelings of worthlessness or guilt resulting in harsh criticism of self.

Clinical depression is diagnosed when several of the above signs and symptoms are present. It is important at this stage to seek medical or therapeutic intervention.

Responding to depression

Working with medication and therapy

Depending on the cause and severity of the depression, medication may be prescribed. Patients should be encouraged to note the effects of the medication and report any side effects (including suicidal thoughts) to their practitioners so other treatment options, alternative medication or therapy can be considered.

Depression recovery programmes

Therapeutic interventions like Dr Neil Nedley's world-renowned depression recovery programme, delivered via books and workbook, DVD or residential setting, has helped thousands in their recovery from depression. More information on these programmes and resources can be accessed at *www.drnedley.com*.

Food factors

A change in eating may occur when individuals experience depression. Lack of appetite, overeating, comfort eating or craving for junk food is common. Essential vitamins and fatty acids are often found to be lacking in the diets of people and are sometimes recommended as supplements for managing the condition.

• Fatty acids make up 15% of the brain's weight. Deficiencies in these nutrients (omega-3 fatty acids) are thought to contribute to severe mental health challenges including depression. Vegetarian sources: flax.

• B vitamins, particularly B6, B9 and B12, are believed to be beneficial for people with depression. Vegetarian sources: B6 – bananas, nuts and seeds, potatoes, whole-grain cereals; B9 – asparagus, nuts, peas, whole grains, yeast; B12 – seaweed, yeast extract.

• Tryptophan is a naturally occurring amino acid used by the body to make serotonin (a brain chemical, affecting mood). Rich sources include bananas and oats.

Exercise

In mild cases of depression, exercise has been found to be as effective as antidepressant drugs in reducing symptoms. Exercise increases the levels of endorphins (happy hormones) which makes you less sensitive to pain and engenders a 'feel good' factor. Exercise enhances health and wellbeing, improves physical appearance, boosts confidence and raises self-esteem. These factors help to improve mood and fight depression. The challenge is the motivation to begin exercising or maintaining it. Gentle encouragement to commence a manageable programme is useful.

Midlife crisis? What is it?

Researcher Nancy Better defines midlife crisis as 'a time of profound psychological turbulence that usually occurs between the ages of 38 and 55, and often results in dramatic life changes. It can last from 2 to 12 years; the defining symptom is a sense that the values that have guided you for many years no longer hold meaning.'

Although many jokes have been made about midlife crises, it is far from amusing to those who suffer debilitating symptoms. It continues to be a controversial syndrome which health experts think is related to the brain or to hormonal changes.

Stages of midlife crisis

It has been found that both males and females go through the same stages during a midlife crisis which mirror the bereavement process.

Shock – Denial – Depression – Anger – Acceptance

What are the key symptoms?

- Irritability

- Lowered self-esteem

- Sudden change in sexual behaviour
  including loss of libido (sex drive)
  or increased sexual appetite

- Erectile dysfunction (impotence)

• Sudden change of image, particularly dressing much younger than one's age in an attempt to look 'youthful'

• Behavioural changes including secrecy, isolation

• Significant change in sleep pattern including insomnia or oversleeping

• Addictive behaviour including significant increase in time spent watching TV, long periods engaged on the Internet

- Fatigue

- Loss of interest in work, family and usual circle of friends

- New circle of friends to the exclusion of former friendships

- Depression characterised by low moods and (often apparently unaccountable) feelings of sadness and lethargy

- Extramarital affairs

Some people have also reported that they have been affected by the following:

- Muscle and joint stiffness

- Night sweats

- Dry skin

- Hair loss

- Weight gain

What causes it?

Unresolved negative experiences and emotions

Some who have had distressing childhood experiences cut themselves off from family members. However, later in life they may feel the need for reconciliation. At this midlife stage they find themselves dealing with deep emotional issues. Unresolved childhood difficulties may cause acute distress, and this realisation can sometimes force the individual to face his own hang-ups and fears, as well as having to learn how to deal with estranged family members. These adjustments take their toll on the emotions.

Working life insecurities

Midlife may be the time when people come to the realisation that they are not going to get to the top of the tree. Accepting this can be hard for some. Additionally, being in a secure position at work in your mid 40s to 50s, but with few promotion prospects, could mean your facing the same routine for the next ten or twenty years.

For others this may be a time when job security becomes more uncertain as companies sometimes dispense with their higher paid, older staff. Facing up to the fact that younger people are being given greater opportunities for promotion could dent the ego. Also if a significant part of someone's life was built around the structure of work and achievement, he might find redundancy or early retirement very difficult.

Health challenges

Coping with illness in midlife can be challenging if the individual has experienced relatively good health up to that point. However, sometimes serious illness may create a powerful urge for change, and it is this change that can sometimes pose a challenge in midlife.

Fears about mortality

Generally, people have a strong desire to deny
their own mortality. However, in midlife we
become increasingly aware that we are
moving towards old age and, inevitably, death.
As we age, people around us die. Losing a
parent, we are pushed into coping with the
pain of loss of a loved one, as well as the
awareness that we are the next generation
and next in line to face death.

Empty nest syndrome

Men as well as women may experience the
'empty nest' syndrome. This is characterised
by the loss or emptiness a parent
feels as children leave home.

It has been found that if either parent has
been too busy pursuing a career to have a
close relationship with the children, he/she may
feel that any chance for a deeper relationship
has slipped past. This gives rise to feelings
of regret, and the impact of the empty
nest can be quite profound.

Marriage break-up

Between the ages of 40 and 60 approximately 30% of marriages dissolve. Numerous reasons are cited. Earlier on, marriages may have been cemented by the shared responsibility of raising children. However when that common purpose no longer exists, this can put a strain on the marriage as attention is focused on their relationship with each other. If the relationship has been unhappy for years, midlife may be the time when individuals feel it's their last chance to commence a new life for themselves.

Other factors may influence the relationship. The power balance in a partnership may change when the roles change. For instance, the husband may find that he has to take early retirement just at the time when his wife is retraining for work, launching out on a new career, developing greater confidence and enjoying greater freedom because the children have left home. The man no longer feels in charge or useful and loses confidence as he is no longer the provider.

Financial challenges

In midlife finances can be affected along with work changes. As individuals move towards retirement or working fewer hours, the financial impact can be significant. This then has an impact on lifestyle and subsequent happiness for some people.

Recessions make people more prone to depression, job insecurity and unemployment. These can adversely affect men's health both physically and in terms of their emotional/mental wellbeing.

Communicating feelings and emotions

The differences in how men and women express thoughts, feelings and emotions can influence the experience of emotional wellbeing. The Mind survey (May 2009) found the following:

- Men were only half as likely as women to talk to their friends about their problems.

- Women were five times more likely to feel tearful than men.

- 45% of men believed they could fight feeling down as opposed to 36% of women.

- 4% of men aged 18-24 years old would see a counsellor if they felt low compared to 13% of women of the same age.

- 37% of men felt worried or low.

- If they felt low for over two weeks only 23% of men would see their GP.

- Men of middle age were seven times more likely than women to have suicidal thoughts.

Gender differences

Nancy Better reports: 'My research shows that women's midlife crises are likely to stem from introspection, a family event, or problem, such as divorce or death or disappointment in their children. Men's midlife crises are more likely to be driven by work or career issues. Even though more women these days are working, I find that these differences haven't entirely disappeared. But men and women alike can be physically reckless, turning to adventure sports or extramarital affairs to deal with midlife angst.'

Numerous reports suggest that men go through midlife crisis because they reach a certain age and realise that life is passing them by. The prevailing emotion tends to be fear:

• Fear of the changes that come with ageing

• Fear of becoming ill

• Fear of becoming less attractive to the opposite sex

• Fear of not attaining goals they have set for themselves

• Fear of dying

Risk factors

Experts suggest that men are more at risk of experiencing symptoms of midlife crisis from the late 30s to age 50. However, some men report symptoms as early as 30 but this is rare. Some psychologists argue that most men go through a midlife crisis to some degree. This they attribute to the fact that all have to deal with what is a time of transition and adjust to a new perspective on life.

What men experience

You may recognise some of the following behaviours and feelings in yourself or other males. Take some time to think about a positive response to each issue and, if necessary, how you can find the appropriate support to assist you.

Psychological triggers

1. He experiences a loss of self-esteem.

2. Challenges on his spiritual journey.
   He questions his faith. He feels
   judged by God and unworthy.

3. Realising he is ageing makes him
   long for the freedom of youth.

Physiological triggers

1. Biological changes. The man realises his body is changing. He begins to lose his hair, his looks, his physique and so on.

2. Lowered testosterone levels cause physical and emotional changes in men. Some argue men go through a male menopause as a result.

3. Trying to recapture his youth or attempting to prevent the inevitable ageing process, he begins dressing younger or returns to youthful styles.

Sociological triggers

1. Work challenges. Work now becomes monotonous. He no longer finds the job exciting. No system or opening for promotion, overlooked for younger employees.

2. Family challenges. He feels trapped in his marriage. His wife and children lose their appeal and he wants to escape from family responsibilities.

Prevalence of midlife crisis

Clinical psychologist Dr Milne states: 'I would guess it affects a significantly small amount of the population. Somewhere around 20% of people (mostly men) will have gone through this by the time they're 50.' He also indicated that everyone's circumstances are different. However, he found that depression made up a significant proportion of midlife crisis.

Is it preventable?

To some degree it is. However, if it occurs due
to sensitivity to hormonal imbalance or falling
levels of testosterone or oestrogen, then
some degree of midlife crisis may be
experienced. However, this can be tempered
by spiritual nurturing, counselling, self-help
techniques and a good holistic lifestyle.

The following tips have been
found to be beneficial:

- **Maintain good health habits**. Avoid the
  temptation to use alcohol, nicotine or
  other drugs as a means of release.

- **De-stressing treatments and exercises**.
  Many complementary approaches, such as
  hydrotherapy, massage and aromatherapy,
  have been found to have a powerful
  relaxing effect.

- **Exercise**. The effects of exercise in promoting positive moods and reducing mild depression are well documented.

- **Prayer**. Having close friends and family pray for you during this time is key to maintaining your emotional and spiritual wellbeing, trust and reliance on God to sustain you at this vulnerable time in your life.

- **Acceptance**. Accept the fact that ageing is a natural process and we all have to face it at some point. We are not immortal.

• **Reassurance.** Life is a journey full of transitions. The journey from youth to middle age and on into old age involves transitions that may seem challenging and uncomfortable. Rather than being fearful, view them as opportunities to re-evaluate and perhaps change the direction of life.

Embrace a positive mindset which captures
the belief that ageing is not simply about
having to give things up, but about new ways
of doing things. When you reach 60, you may
well be only two-thirds or less of the way
through your life. With a good lifestyle, even
centenarians are now enjoying quality of life.
With so much of life left yet to be experienced,
it leaves a time to broaden your interests,
travel, return to education, learn new
work skills or take up new sports.

Do I need to see a doctor?

It may be necessary to seek medical help if there are significant health or physiological changes. Additionally, if you are emotionally fragile an assessment may also be useful. If you feel you'd like to talk your problems over with a sympathetic stranger, such as a counsellor, your GP can refer you. There are also very helpful Christian counsellors who will help you while encouraging you to maintain your spiritual wellbeing. Never be afraid to ask for help.

Self-help/Alternative treatments

• **Increase B vitamins.** A daily dose of a B complex is useful. This assists in testosterone production, boosts energy and enhances blood flow to the sexual organs.

• **Maintain zinc levels.** Research demonstrates that men low in zinc have low testosterone, low sex drive and a low sperm count. Smoking, alcohol and coffee deplete zinc levels. Take multivitamin and mineral supplements that contain zinc.

Maintain as wholesome and natural a diet as possible. Eliminate junk foods as they aggravate stress symptoms.

Regular exercise. This releases endorphins and gives a positive 'feel good' factor.

Christian counselling. This encourages expression and assists in addressing issues.

Conclusion

There are many facets to good health –
physical, emotional, spiritual and social. While
we have not been able to cover all the
research in these areas, we have endeavoured
to look at the major issues relating to male
health. As we come to the close of this book
of health for men, here are some key pointers
to follow to ensure a wholesome balanced life
and assist in your pursuit of wellbeing.

- Take up regular health screening available in relation to your age.

- Exercise regularly to improve circulation, co-ordination and balance.

- Increase vegetable protein like beans and lentils in place of meat.

- Replace saturated fats with unsaturated fats.

- Include at least 4 servings of pulses in your diet weekly.

- Eat at least one tablespoon of nuts or seeds every day.

- Drink 2 litres of water daily to boost brain function and keep skin healthy.

- Manage stress effectively.

- Have a balanced life with adequate rest and sleep.

- Nurture faith and trust in God, have an active prayer life and keep a positive attitude to encourage good spiritual and mental health.

- Avoid exposure to toxins.

- Watch for any signs of bodily changes and seek medical assessment.

- Enjoy social interaction with family and friends.

- Be happy! Find one thing each day for which you are grateful and give thanks for it!

So there you have it. Some key 'must dos' for holistic health. May you enjoy the journey to wellness as you embrace these principles of health and good living!